MW01504178

WAKING UP TO 5G

THE INVISIBLE WORLD OF
FREQUENCIES
and
STEPS TO TAKE NOW TO PREPARE

BARBARA J. SCHNEIDER MS
DR. PATRICIA L. YODER

1

This book details the authors' personal experiences with and opinions about 5G. The authors are not your healthcare providers.

The author and publisher are providing this book and its contents on an "as is" basis and make no representations or warranties of any kind with respect to this book or its contents.

The statements made about 5G, products and services have not been evaluated by the U.S. Food and Drug administration. They are not intended to diagnose, treat, cure, or prevent any condition or disease. Please consult with your own physician or healthcare specialist regarding the suggestions and recommendations made in this book.

Except as specifically stated in this book, neither the author or publisher, nor any authors, contributors, or other representatives will be liable for damages arising out of or in connection with the use of this book.

This is a comprehensive limitation of liability that applies to all damages of any kind, including (without
limitation) compensatory; direct, indirect or consequential damages; loss of data, income or profit; loss of or damage to property and claims of third parties.

As such, use of this book implies your acceptance of this disclaimer

TABLE OF CONTENTS

Chapter 1.
What is 5G?
Chapter 2.
Low Frequency Electric Fields
Chapter 3.
Brain Frequencies
Chapter 4.
Our Bodies Speak in Frequencies
Chapter 5.
Smart Meters
Chapter 6.
5G Technologies
Chapter 7
Take Preventative action
Chapter 8.
Tips for a Healthy Immune System
Chapter 9.
Stress
Chapter 10.
Summing It Up

Introduction

We live in a world that vibrates with frequencies. A frequency is the number of repeating vibrations that occur in a second. Frequencies are measured in hertz (Hz). Everything vibrates with a particular frequency; even the human body.

We also live in a world of electronic devices that make our lives easier, more productive, and entertaining. Looking around we can see people carrying smart phones, electric tablets, computers, wearing smart watches and utilizing a plethora of other available "smart" devices. This world of visable conveniences rely on an invisible world of frequencies.

Exposure to electromagnetic fields is nothing new. However as the demand for electricity and advanced technologies have increased, environmental exposure to man-made electromagnetic fields is rising rapidly. Daily, everyone is exposed to a mixture of complex magnetic and electric fields, both at work and home. There is no way to avoid it; especially now that we have been promised 5G technology everywhere on earth, even rural areas.

The human body has vibrational frequency down to the cellular level. It carries tiny electrical currents due to normal chemical reactions that are a part of normal bodily functions even when there is no exposure to man-made electromagnetic fields. Our heart, nerves, digestion, brain, in fact, every organ in our body rely on signals and react biochemically to the rearrangement of charged particles.

We are now faced with the invisible appearance of 5G which is the next generation of mobile broadband.

Since there are more questions than answers, the focus of this book is to educate the general population of both the advantages and hazards of the "Invisible World of 5G" and the affect it may have on our physical and mental health.

We are in not trying to alarm you or raise fear. Our simple intention is to make the reader aware of 5g frequencies and encourage further research on the subject.

CHAPTER 1.

WHAT IS 5G?

5G stands for fifth-generation cellular wireless. It is also used simultaneously for millimeter waves. For the purpose of this book, we will use the term 5G for both fifth-generation cellular and 5GHz. Initially, at the end of 2017, there was a set of standards created for it. Those standards have changed and what we have now is an ominous web of confusion.

5G is not simply a fast and furious wave of broadband that allows users to use the internet at lightning speed. As it stands now there are three main forms of 5G. In the future we will see larger channels (in order to speed up the flow of data), lower latency (to bring about responsiveness and prevent lag), and the ability to connect many devices at one time.

5G can run on any frequency which enables three multifarious experiences: low, middle, and high. The width of each available channel and how many channels are available is related directly to the speed of **5G**. In low band the width is narrow, and the channels are few, there are more available in mid-band and in high band there are many. High band contains an immense number of unused airwaves, which is difficult for carriers to work with. What makes 5G so reliable is its adaptability to switch beams. A 5G phone will continuously monitor its signal quality when it is connected to a high frequency (millimeter wave) band. It constantly keeps searching for other reliable signals. If the 5G phone detects its signal is about to become unreliable it smoothly switches over to a new frequency band until it finds a faster more reliable connection. This prevents lag when watching videos, making video calls, live streaming, or downloading apps or videos (Segan, 2020).

Band Frequencies

Low band 5 G frequencies operate in frequencies below 1GHz. These frequencies can travel great distances but there are few wide channels available. Many of the channels that are available are used for 4G.

Mid-band 5G frequencies operate in the 1-10GHz range. This is the range (at the time of this writing) that most of the cellular and Wi-Fi frequencies operate in. Users of these networks create range from the towers.

High-band 5G, or millimeter-wave, operates in the 20-100GHz range (Heinzman, 2019). Millimeter-wave spectrum is usually defined to include frequencies between 30GHz and 300GHz. But in the context of 5G, carriers and regulators have generally targeted frequencies between 24GHz and 90GHz (Brodkin, 2019). T-Mobile's high-frequency spectrum includes licenses in the 28GHz and 39GHz bands. These airwaves haven't been used for consumer applications before and are very short range. Tests show that these waves will travel about 800 feet. The waves may be short but are mostly unused. These millimeter-wave signals drop off faster than those at a lower frequency and because they transfer such an enormous amount of data, more landline internet connections will be required. This will require cellular providers to implement an abundant amount of smaller, lower-powered base stations outputting about 2-10 watts in order to offer the multi-gigabit speeds that they are promising.

These small cells have already been installed in major cities to increase 4G capacity. All that needs to be done to bring it up to **5G** speed is bolt an extra radio onto the existing site (Heinzman, 2019).

5G Cellular VS 5GHz or "5G E"

Many individuals are confused and think 5G is the same as millimeter-wave, (the very short-range, high-speed frequency promising lightning speed). Because the millimeter-wave has a problem with penetrating walls and traveling long distances, what we are seeing the carriers install (at the time of this writing) is fifth generation cell phone networks. Wi- Fi 5G can run on any frequency which enables three multifarious experiences: low, middle and high. When referring to Wi-Fi; "5G(Hz) is a frequency band of five gigahertz. When referring to cellular; 5G stands for generation. The terms are completely different. The industry has settled on 5G NR "new radio" as the standard technology. Carriers do not need the millimeter-wave to install what they deem as 5G. They can install it on existing 4G frequencies. For example 600 MHz to 3 GHz (Ultra High

Frequency, UHF) and even up to 6 GHz, as well as millimeter wave bands 24 to 86 GHz (Super High Frequency to Extremely High Frequency). Using these frequencies, they can use the same towers as 4G with lower lag and greater speed (Segan, 2020).

Are Millimeter Wave Bands Safe?

Proponents state the millimeter waves are safe "but should be monitored". Opponents demand that the waves be proven safe before it is deployed. According to IEEE Senior Member David Witkowski, cochair of the initiative's Deployment Working Group, " Showering, cooking breakfast, commuting to work, eating in a restaurant, being out in public— everything we do carries risk," he says. "Whether we're talking about 3G, 4G, or 5G, the question of electromagnetic radiation safety (EMR) is whether the risks are manageable (Pretz, 2019).

12

Citing this large body of research, more than 240 scientists who have published peer-reviewed research on the biological and health effects of nonionizing electromagnetic fields (EMF) signed the International EMF Scientist Appeal, which calls for stronger exposure limits. The appeal makes the following claims:

"Numerous recent scientific publications have shown that EMF affects living organisms at levels well below most international and national guidelines. Effects include increased cancer risk, cellular stress, increase in harmful free radicals, genetic damages, structural and functional changes of the reproductive system, learning and memory deficits, neurological disorders, and negative impacts on general well-being in humans. Damage goes well beyond the human race, as there is growing evidence of harmful effects to both plant and animal life."

The scientists who signed this appeal arguably constitute the majority of experts on the effects of nonionizing radiation. They have published more than 2,000 papers and letters on EMF in professional journals.

"The FCC's RFR (radio frequency radiation) exposure limits regulate the intensity of exposure, taking into account the frequency of the carrier waves, but ignore the signaling properties of the RFR. Along with the patterning and duration of exposures, certain characteristics of the signal (e.g., pulsing, polarization) increase the biologic and health impacts of the exposure. New exposure limits are needed which account for these differential effects. Moreover, these limits should be based on a biological effect, not a change in a laboratory rat's behavior."

"The World Health Organization's International Agency for Research on Cancer (IARC) classified RFR as "possibly carcinogenic to humans" in 2011. Last year, a $30 million study conducted by the U.S. National Toxicology Program (NTP) found "clear evidence" that two years of exposure to cell phone RFR increased cancer in male rats and damaged DNA in rats and mice of both sexes. The Ramazzini Institute in Italy replicated the key finding of the NTP using a different carrier frequency and much weaker exposure to cell phone radiation over the life of the rat." (Moskowitz, 2019)

Trump's 2020 Executive Order

President Trump issued an executive order on March 25, 2020 "The National Strategy to Secure 5G". The following is from his announcement:

Facilitating domestic 5G rollout;
Assessing the risks and identifying core security principles for 5G infrastructure; (in the announcement

the "risks" have to do with security not health risks.)
Managing the risks to our economic and national security from the use of 5G infrastructure.

And

Promoting responsible global development and deployment of 5G infrastructure (The United States will emphasize the need for open and transparent processes to develop timely, technically robust, and appropriate standards. The United States will promote and support increased participation by the private sector and ensure that such participation is informed by appropriate public-private coordination.)

The announcement also states:
"Criminals and foreign adversaries will seek to steal information transiting the networks for monetary gain and

16

exploit these systems and devices for intelligence collection and surveillance. Adversaries may also disrupt or maliciously modify the public and private services that rely on communications infrastructure. Given these threats, 5G infrastructure must be secure and reliable to maintain information security and address risks to critical infrastructure, public health and safety, and economic and national security." (Vincent, 2020).

Once the executive order is published it can be read in its entirety at https://www.federalregister.gov/pres idential-documents/executive-orders/donald-trump/2020

THE RISKS BEING REPORTED

We do not want to spread fear. It is our desire to help everyone be aware of what could happen to their bodies in a **5G** world and provide information on how to support the immune system as well as other precautionary measures.

Following are **some** of the risks that
are being reported:

- **Cancer Risks**
- **Immune problems**
- **Cellular Stress**
- **Increase in harmful free radicals**
- **Genetic damages**
- **Structural and functional changes of the reproductive system**
- **Learning and memory deficits**
- **Neurological disorders** (Moskowitz, 2019)
- **Skin Problems** - An Israeli study on 5G frequencies found that they cause human sweat ducts to behave strangely. A study particularly focused on the skin feared 5G frequency of 60 GHz, (referenced by the Center for Public Integrity)concluded that "more than 90% of the transmitted (MMWs) power is absorbed in

18

the epidermis and dermis layer." It appears **5G** is not going to be good for the skin, it would appear.

- **Heart Problems** - A study from 1992 reported that frequencies in the higher 5G spectrum, ranging from 53-78GHz could probably cause heart arrhythmia in humans.

- **Eye Problems** - In 1994, a study was carried out in Poland found that low level millimeter wave radiation could cause human beings to develop eye problems and cataracts. Also, a Japanese experiment found that "millimeter-wave antennas can cause thermal injuries of varying types of levels. The thermal effects induced by millimeter waves can apparently penetrate below the surface of the eye." (Johnson, 2018)

- **Mental Health Problems**

What About Nature?

We are already destroying nature because of our use of technology, as revealed in an analysis from EKLIPSE, which discerned over 97 studies, confirms that electromagnetic radiation from cell towers as well as power lines disorientate birds and insects. They also destroy the health of plants. The analysis warns that 5G will increase the threat to plants, birds and insects. The findings are not new. There have been many reports over the last decade supporting these findings.

Exposure to electromagnetic radiation disturbs the natural orientation and navigation mechanisms of bees and other insects, who use the earth's magnetic field and light energy to orient and navigate. It makes them restless, develop an urge to swarm, increasingly aggressive, and colony collapse in 62.5% of apiaries.

The UK charity "Buglife" states that plans for installing 5G will cause serious impacts on the environment and suggests transmitters not be placed on LED streetlamps that attract insects. The charity is calling for further study. (Dovey, 2020)

Researchers testing 5G millimeter waves, have discovered rain is susceptible to absorbing the radiation. As water falls from the sky, scientists fear plants can be contaminated with radiation and ultimately become inedible. In 2010, a study on aspen seedlings determined exposure to radio frequencies caused leaves to exhibit necrosis symptoms, while Armenian-based trials revealed low-intensity millimeter waves invoke peroxidase (a stress protein in plants) and isoenzyme spectrum changes of wheat shoots.

Since 2000, there have been documented instances of radiation sources (like cell towers) causing birds to abandon their nests, along with experiencing health issues like plumage deterioration, locomotion problems, and reduced survivorship. Non-ionizing microwave radiation has also been linked to declining bee populations, which reduce a queen's egg-laying capabilities. A 2012 Loyola College study concluded that out of 919 research studies conducted on birds, plants, bees, humans, and other animals, 593 subjects showed signs of being affected by RF-EMG radiation.

Property Values

Once 5G is deployed widespread there will be thousands of small cell towers popping up in our neighborhoods. Some will be in our front and back yards. In addition to health concerns, many homeowners are nervous about declining property values. A study by the National Association of Realtors disclosed homes located in proximity of cellphone towers are declining in value. Some properties dropped 20-30 percent.

Not only will there be many more cell towers, they will be closer together. Projections from experts divulged telecommunication conglomerates will need 400 small towers to cover the uptown section of a city the size of Charlotte, North Carolina and almost 28,000 to expand across a whole area of a city that size. Because **5G** doesn't travel as far as our current wireless frequencies, the towers will be required to be approximately 100-500 yards apart. One way to cover the towers up is the use of "small cell" sites disguising them to look like streetlights, utility poles, trees, cactus and any other type of objects.

MIMO

The miniaturization of base stations also enables another technological breakthrough for **5G**: Massive MIMO. MIMO stands for multiple-input multiple-output and refers to a configuration that takes advantage of the smaller antennas needed for millimeter waves by dramatically increasing the number of antenna ports in each base station.

Harish Krishnaswamy, associate professor of electrical engineering at Columbia University stated, "With a massive number of antennas — tens to hundreds of antennas at each base station — you can serve many different users at the same, increasing the data rate,". At the Columbia high-Speed and Millimeter-wave IC (COSMIC) lab, Krishnaswamy and his team designed chips that enable both millimeter wave and MIMO technologies. "Millimeter-wave and massive MIMO are the two biggest technologies **5G** will use to deliver the higher data rates and lower latency we expect to see."

Massive MIMO is a key enabler of **5G's** extremely fast data rates and promises to raise **5G's** potential to a new level. The primary benefits of massive MIMO to the network and end users can be summed up as:

Increased Network Capacity – Network Capacity is defined as the total data volume that can be served to a user and the maximum number of levels of expected service. Massive MIMO contributes to increased capacity first by enabling **5G** NR deployment in the higher frequency range in Sub-6 GHz (e.g., 3.5 GHz); and second by employing MU-MIMO where multiple users are served with the same time and frequency resources.

Improved Coverage – With massive MIMO, users enjoy a more uniform experience across the network, even at the cell's edge – so users can expect high data rate service almost everywhere. Moreover, 3D beamforming enables dynamic coverage required for moving users (e.g., users traveling in cars or connected cars) and adjusts the coverage to suit user location, even in locations that have relatively weak network coverage.

User experience – Ultimately, the above two benefits result in a better overall user experience — users can transfer large data files or download movies, or use data-hungry apps on the go, wherever life takes them.

As mentioned earlier, MIMO has been used in wireless communications for many years. But now, in the context of **5G** NR, massive MIMO is radically changing how and when we choose to use our mobile devices. We no longer have to second guess if we're in a good area to download or transfer large files. The user experience is about to take an immense leap forward.

Massive MIMO can offer enhanced broadband services in the future, and more. **5G** networks are expected to support a great variety of wireless services in areas ranging from infotainment to healthcare, smart homes and cities, manufacturing, and many others. Location awareness in wireless networks may enable many applications such as emergency services, autonomous driving and geographic routing. Massive MIMO technology can be tailored to support a massive number of Massive Machine Type Communication (MTC) devices. Also, it is an excellent candidate to realize Ultra Reliable Communication as it can establish very robust physical links

First responders who often operate in chaotic, changing situations and can't rely on cellular networks or other existing fixed infrastructure to be operational when needed due to natural disasters, power outages, overloaded networks, or other issues will find MIMO as an advantage.

Broadcast television production, such as live sports or news broadcasts, where the story may change during broadcast and video transmission locations have to move without notice, or where the shoot might involve multiple, simultaneous areas of interest. MIMO will eliminate long, expensive cable runs.

MIMO technology will come to the aid of law enforcement or military users who need to operate their own separate communication networks on dedicated radio bands. This includes intra-team communication among small groups, as well as larger networks that include ground vehicles, UAV / UGV systems, and more.

Opponents to massive MIMO believe it is attractive to terrorist and vulnerable to cyber-attacks because governments, will be able to collect more detailed data across geographies and, with the help of algorithms, predict and respond immediately to emergencies such as pandemics or extreme weather events. Combining 5G with mobile apps, sensors, internet-of-things devices, and predictive algorithms could turn notoriously slow

28

local governments into well-oiled operators, with tools that span traffic, safety, and city services.

There's no question that such a high level of surveillance and data capture comes with privacy risks--a particularly important issue in U.S. cities. It is necessary to plan now on how to protect citizens' privacy while advancing new technologies that help them. Before long the network will ultimately pave the way for truly connected smart cities that could be taken down easily in a cyber-attack.

There are big risks beyond privacy. When things fail--and they will--they could fail spectacularly. Hackers will hit the mother lode, as they'll be able to siphon off dramatically more sensitive data far faster than they ever could before. Cybersecurity will only grow more important and the cybersecurity industry will have to grow to accommodate it. Think about 5.8

billion IoT devices next year, ranging from remote robotic surgeons to autonomous vehicles. It's one thing to hack someone's doorbell, but another to hack into an autonomous vehicle or a hospital's medical devices.

Is 5G A Weapon?

"Access to the 5G-millimeter wave bandwidth will be critical to operations in all war-fighting domains, in particular, space command & control"

A widely interviewed inventor of Head of display and battlefield interrogation weapons mitigation, Mark Steele, won a victory in the fight against 5G , when a court in Britain upheld the right of people to know the dangers of unproven 5G microwave technology. Gateshead, UK Recorder Nolan QC refused to "gag" Mr. Steele who has been very outspoken and has stated in numerous interviews that **5G** operating in the 24-100GHz rang is actually sub-gigahertz which means it is under the GHz threshold, so still measured in MHz). He claims **5G** is a weapons system much like long-range radar and directed energy (know as DEW and was used in 9/11 and various fires). He suggests that when **5G** hardware is examined, a dielectric lens can be detected which proves it is a weapons system. He also states that it is powerful enough to kill babies in the wombs. According to Steele, autonomous vehicles can use **5G** to shine in the mirrors of other drivers. Quoting from Mr. Steele, "**5G** is a weapons system, nothing more, nothing less. It's got nothing to do with telecommunications for humans. 5G is a machine to machine connection for autonomous vehicles." (Westall, 2020). It has also been said that **5G** uses the exact frequencies used by the military for their non-lethal weapons such as

Active Denial Systems for crowd dispersal. These weapons have the capacity to cause tremendous injury. One Dr. states that if you are in a crowed being dispersed using this technology, your body will feel like it is on fire.

Proponents of massive MIMO state that it will be a great help to soldiers on the battlefield, although jamming is a concern.

The possibilities offered by this new technology are explained by the Defense Applications of **5G** Network Technology, published by the Defense Science Board, a federal committee which provides scientific advice for the Pentagon: "The emergence of 5G technology, now commercially available, offers the Department of Defense the opportunity to take advantage, at minimal cost, of the benefits of this system for its own operational requirements".

That means, the **5G** commercial network, built and activated by private companies, will be used by the U.S. armed forces at a much lower expenditure than that necessary if the network were to be set up with an exclusively military goal. Military experts foresee that the **5G** system will play an essential role for the use of hypersonic weapons – missiles, including those bearing nuclear warheads, which travel at a speed superior to Mach 5 (five times the speed of sound). In order to guide the missiles on variable trajectories, changing direction in a fraction of a second to avoid interceptor missiles, it is necessary to gather, elaborate and transmit enormous quantities of data in a very short time. The same thing is necessary to activate defenses in case of an attack with this type of weapon – since there is not enough time to take such decisions, the only possibility is to rely on **5G** automatic systems.

This new technology will also play a key role in the battle network. With the capability of simultaneously linking millions of transceivers within a defined area, it will enable military personnel – departments and individuals – to transmit to one another, almost in real time, maps, photos and other information about the operation under way.

5G will also be extremely important for the secret services and special forces. It will enable control and espionage systems which are far more efficient than those we use today. It will improve the lethality of killer drones and war robots by giving them the capacity of identifying, following and targeting people based on facial recognition and other characteristics. The **5G** network, as a weapon of high-tech capacity, will also become the target for cyber-attacks and war actions carried out with new generation weapons (Dinucci, 2019).

EMP and HPM Attacks and 5G

Back in 2018 the Washington Examiner wrote "Military warns EMP attack could wipe out America, 'democracy, world order'". In early 2019 President Trump signed an executive order meant to protect the United States from an EMP, directing federal agencies to coordinate in assessing, planning and guarding against its risks from human and natural sources.

An EMP (Electro Magnetic Pulse) is a high-intensity surge of energy that can disrupt or destroy electronics by, essentially, overloading them. There are two ways an EMP could potentially pose a large-scale threat to U.S. security.

The first is through the detonation of a nuclear warhead at high altitude. We know this because, in 1962, the U.S. tested a nuclear bomb 250 miles above the Pacific Ocean. The test led to electronic disturbance 900 miles away in Hawaii. Specifically, streetlights were blown out, telephones went dead, and U.S., British and Soviet satellites were damaged.

The second is through a natural solar superstorm, known as a geomagnetic disturbance (GMD), which has about a 10 percent chance of occurring every decade, according to NASA. An event like this took place in 1859 and caused telegraph circuits to catch on fire.

A congressional report states "The threat of an EMP attack against the United States is hard to assess, but some observers indicate that it is growing along with worldwide access to newer technologies". It also said, "... a single, specially designed low-yield

36

nuclear explosion high above the United States, or over a battlefield, can produce a large-scale EMP effect that could result in a widespread loss of electronics, but no direct fatalities, and may not necessarily evoke a large nuclear retaliatory strike by the U.S. military."

5G technologies and access to **5G** spectrum are crucial to not only democratic and economic interests but also communications and other war operations, such as may be in effect during an EMP-attack scenario, especially command and control. In effect, control of **5G** is both control of the Internet and control of the future war landscape.

Following are some of the damages associated with an EMP:

- TVs, radios and other broadcast equipment

- Power grid transformers and substations
- Telephones (land lines) and mobile phones
- Vehicle and aircraft control systems
- Computers and all internet connected devices
- Refrigerators
- Generators
- Satellites potentially within the range of the EMP
- Anything electronic or powered by electricity could be damaged by an EMP. The damage will vary with the size of the EMP and how close you are to the center of the energy from the EMP.

The same report reveals, HPM weapons are smaller in scale, and can sometimes involve a much lower level of technology, which may be within the capability of some extremist groups or non-state organizations.

HPM (high-power microwaves) can cause damage to computers similar to HEMP (High Electromagnetic Pulse), although the effects are limited to a much smaller area. The technical accessibility, lower cost, and the apparent vulnerability of U.S. civilian electronic equipment could make small-scale HPM weapons attractive for terrorist groups in the future.

DE (Directed Energy) weapons, lasers, and other EMS phenomena are often undetectable until the effects are encountered. However, once the effects are encountered, it may be too late to mitigate harmful effects. Consequently, in the future, unmanned aircraft, ships, and other vehicles may be preferable to manned defense mechanisms.

Physical and Biological Impacts

Symptoms include and are not limited to:

- Fatigue
- Nausea
- Severe headache
- Warming sensation of the skin and body
- Skin erythema and pain
- Heat stress to eye lens
- Concussion like symptoms
- Dizziness
- Sleep problems
- Loss of hearing

As events in Cuba and China demonstrated, personnel can become ill from EMS effects. Although the nature of EMS activities that caused health issues for more than 20 diplomats is not entirely understood, what is well understood are the effects. In short, personnel at those locations are believed to have suffered traumatic brain injury (while in bed sleeping).

The victims had reported hearing intense high-pitched sounds in their hotel rooms or homes followed by symptoms like nausea, severe headaches, fatigue, dizziness, sleep problems and loss of hearing. A senior administration official stated investigator checked the hotel rooms and homes but did not find any acoustic devices. This led law enforcement to believe the injuries were a result of microwaves beamed from a nearby location. The "sounds" were a means of hiding the microwave attacks. The official said this was only a theory and there was no concrete evidence to prove it. Brain scans showed changes that indicated damage.

Beatrice Golomb, a professor of medicine at the University of California, San Diego, agreed with Smith. "Reported facts appear consistent with pulsed (radio frequency/microwave radiation) as the source of injury in Cuba diplomats. Non-diplomats citing symptoms from RF/MW ... report compatible health conditions," she said in a paper slated for publication later this month.

"The specifics of the varied sounds that the diplomats reported hearing during the apparent inciting episodes, such as chirping, ringing and buzzing, cohere in detail with known properties of so-called 'microwave hearing,' also known as the Frey effect," she said in university news release.

The U.S. State Department issued a statement neither confirming nor denying the possibility of microwave attack (Vaidyanatha, 2018).

Will We Become Human Antennas?

A study by researcher Arthur Firstenberg, was published in 2002. In his analysis he explains the electromagnetic pulses from 5G replicate inside the human body to create tiny new internal **5G** antennas. He states that the re-radiated waves are named Brillouin Precursors. Firstenberg states "This means that the reassurance we are being given – that these millimeter waves are too short to penetrate far into the body – is not true." (Freeman, 2020)

5G From Space

There are plans to beam 5G from space. At least five companies are requesting permission to provide 5G from space using a combination of 20,000 satellites placed in low and medium orbits above the earth. The beams from these satellites will be steerable. In example, metal particulates sprayed in chemtrails can be used by **5G**.

Another environmental concern comes from **5G** satellites, which have shorter lifespans, and will require more frequent launches than we currently see. A new type of hydrocarbon engine is expected to power these suborbital rocket fleets, which would emit black carbon and other hazardous substances like chlorine into the atmosphere. According to one Californian study, these emission rates could potentially cause significant changes in global atmospheric circulation, along with ozone and temperature distributions.

According to an article in *Radiation Health Risks,* Governments and other global entities are behind the roll out of **5G** for more reasons than just increasing data capacities for civilian communications. **5G** has huge military uses and functions. Some of you may have heard or remember US President Donald J Trump creating the new U.S. "Space Force". Well he is talking about **5G** technology.

China developed a space technology using "Quantum Entanglement". This technology uses satellites and enables military communication that surpasses anything we have ever had or used in human history. China had a satellite that launched in August of 2016 which has now validated across a record 1200 kilometers using the "spooky action" that Albert Einstein said he abhorred. In the test of China's satellite, entangled photons were sent to separate stations on earth. Measuring one photon's quantum state instantly determines the other, no matter how far away it is. And then they pair. One Photon can be sent to a particular station on earth while the other photon, it's pair, remains in the satellite. When a third photon is entangled with the one on earth this is communicated back to the satellite. This enables a new encrypted method of communication. So basically, what Quantum Entanglement is a way for a military to communicate amongst

45

themselves in a way that is extremely difficult for an enemy to crack. (It also gives that nation the ability to more easily decode enemy encrypted communications.) It is an encrypted form of communication that we did not even think was possible. Albert Einstein thought of it in theory. China is developing this attempting to set up a space-based military communication system that will not be able to be cracked by its enemies

Symptoms

Current electromagnetic frequencies may cause and not limited to the following symptoms caused by current electromagnetic frequencies:

- Headache
- Fatigue
- Decreased ability to concentrate
- Tinnitus
- Irritability
- Insomnia

- Heart problems
- Nervous system challenges
- Intense body heat and pain
- Immune system abnormalities
- Cancer
- Birth defects
- DNA changes (NTD, 2019)

The Bottom Line

Our position is neither for nor against **5G.** What we are saying is that it is time to educate the public about what is good about **5G** and the possibility of it harming us. Many individuals want lightning fast download speeds, and the marvels of driverless cars, remote medical procedures, and other new technology. At the same time our heath is of utmost importance. We only know about the risks that have been studied. We watched the government hearings where doctors pleaded that more studies must be done before it is released. Erin Brockovich has joined the fight against 5G along with many other groups and individuals.

We suggest that you educate yourself before the rollout, in order to be prepared. As the saying goes, "Hope for the best, prepare for the worse".

CHAPTER 2.

LOW FREQUENCY ELECTRIC FIELDS

Because the human body is made up of charged particles, low frequency electric fields such as 5G create an influence on all of us. Just as any material made up of charged particles react to low frequency electric fields by current flowing through the material to the ground, magnetic fields induce circulating currents within our bodies. The stronger the intensity of the magnetic field, the stronger the currents within our bodies. Large enough currents can cause nerves and muscles to be stimulated or affect other biological processes (World Health Organization, 2019).

Infrasound

Our world can be noisy and loud. It is commonly known that loud noises can cause hearing damage. What is not commonly known, is in the invisible frequency world there are damaging noises that we cannot hear. Humans cannot usually hear sounds below 20 hertz. There are animals that communicate in this range, but infrasound is often artificial coming from public address systems, industrial machinery, loudspeakers and other devices. Studies show that sound around 7hz can produce nausea, dizziness, migraines, fatigue and tinnitus with no attributable cause.

The definition of infrasound is any sound lower than 20 hertz, which is the normal limit of hearing for a human being. Experiments have brought forth information that infrasound can produce a wide and strange range of effects in those who experience it, including anxiety, shivers, and extreme

50

sorrow. In general, humans cannot consciously perceive infrasound, but they can feel it. In a British study, researchers played music laced with infrasound for test subjects, and 22 percent reported feelings of uneasiness, revulsion, or fear after listening (McPhilips, 2015).

Also, researchers have indicated that infrasound may be responsible for "feeling creepy and spooky". As a matter of fact, the 18.9 HZ range has been dubbed the "fear frequency". According to British engineer, Vic Tandy this frequency can cause feelings of depression, the occasional cold shiver and the visual appearance of ghostly figures. He came to this deduction when he noticed some odd events in his lab. A colleague who was sitting at a desk experienced the symptoms and thought Tandy was standing at his side, only to realize that he was across the room. Everyone was very busy, so paid little attention to the event, until one-night Tandy was working alone at the desk and started to sweat although he was cold, and the cats were moving around strangely. He felt as if there was something in the room with him. He looked around the lab checking on everything, including leaks in the gas bottles. Everything was in order, so he returned to the desk. Once again, he felt as if he was being watched. Slowly a figure emerged from the left, it was on the periphery of his vision and indistinct, yet it moved as a person would. The figure was silent and its coloring grey. This made the hair on Mr. Tandy's neck stand up and he felt a chill in the room. He later admitted that he was terrified. When he finally gathered up the courage to face the apparition it faded and disappeared. He had no evidence to support what he had seen and experienced. He decided he was "cracking up" and went home. The following day, he went back to cut a thread into a foil blade. Five minutes into the job, he left the blade in the vice to fetch a drop of oil to make the job easier. Upon his return, found the free end of the blade vibrating up and down. He immediately began to feel a twinge of fright. Because the vibrating pieces of metal were familiar to him, unlike the apparition he saw before, he decided to experiment. He realized the vibrating blade was receiving energy which must have been varying in intensity and at a rate equal to the resonant frequency of the blade. In most cases this type of energy is referred to as sound. Although, there was background noise there must have been sound that he could not hear. Tandy, place the blade in a drill vice and slid it along the floor. The vibration increased until the blade was level with the desk, which was half-way down the room, after passing the desk it reduced in amplitude and entirely stopped when it reached the end of the room. Mr. Tandy and his assistants were sharing their lab with a low frequency standing wave. The wave was at the exact frequency to enable it to be reflected back by the walls at each end of the lab so it could not go anywhere, therefore it was a standing wave. The wave, in effect, was folded back on itself reinforcing the peak energy in the center of the room. Tandy calculated the frequency as 18.98Hz (Tandy, 1998).

There are many sources of infrasound including, storms, earthquakes, animals, winds, and manmade devices. In example, elephants use infrasound to communicate over long distances; since low frequency sounds travel farther than high frequency ones, infrasound is ideal for communicating from far away. These communications, or "rumbles," were discovered by a researcher who felt, rather than heard, the elephants rumbling to each other. The discovery of elephant rumblings offers a solution to the question of how elephant families can coordinate patterns of movement when separated, and how males find far-away females for breeding. Whales also use infrasonic sound, and have been observed communicating with each other over distances of hundreds of miles (McPhilips, 2015)

When it comes to regulating infrasound, the bad news is guidelines are outdated and the guidelines that are in place are not strong enough. Workplace exposure to infrasound as well as ultrasound usually exceed current guidelines. More research needs to be done regarding what is safe.

INFRASOUND AND THE HUMAN BODY

Our bodies can generate infrasonic waves. It is known that the human body can generate mechanical vibrations at very low frequencies, so-called infrasonic waves. Such low-frequency vibrations are generated by physiological processes—heartbeats, respiratory movements, blood flow in vessels, and other processes. Each organ in the human body produces a different resonance frequency. The heart resonance frequency is ~ 1 hz. The brain has a resonance frequency of ~ 10 hz, blood circulation about 0.05 to 0.3 hz. (National Research Nuclear University, 2016) .

CHAPTER 3.

BRAIN FREQUENCIES

When we enter a hospital or an airplane, we are asked to turn off our cellphones. That is because the electromagnetic transmissions they emit can interfere with sensitive electrical devices. Our brain is also a sensitive electric device. Neuron transmitted bioelectricity which is transmitted inside our skull create all our thoughts and sensations. Electric fields generated between neurons radiate out of brain tissue as electrical waves. These waves can be measured in EEGs by placing electrodes on an individual's scalp. "So fundamental are brainwaves to the internal workings of the mind, they have become the ultimate legal definition drawing the line between life and death (Fields, 2008).

Scientists have also been able to use transcranial magnetic stimulation (TMS) to selectively control brain function. TMS uses powerful pulses of electromagnetic radiation beamed into an individual's brain to alter its circuitry.

Could **5G** technology operating in resonance with the brain's frequencies affect our brainwaves? Studies have revealed that cellphones although not as powerful as TMS do affect our brainwaves (Fields, 2008).

We all have brain wave frequencies. There are four categories: Alpha, Beta, Delta, and Theta.

Brain Wave Frequencies:

DELTA (0.1 to 3.5 Hz)
Delta are the lowest frequencies of the brain and occur during deep sleep and processes that are abnormal. The delta frequencies are dominant in infants until they are about a year old. When Delta waves are increased, our real-

world awareness is decreased. Also, we access information in our unconscious mind through the Delta often severely restricts the ability to focus and maintain attention. It is as if the brain is locked into a perpetual drowsy state (Neurohealth, 2020).

In a study conducted by James Horne at Loughborough University Sleep Research Centre in England, it was found that cell phone signals alter an individual's behavior during the call and continued long after the phone was turned off. Some of the test subjects had trouble falling asleep. Using a basic cell phone (Nokia 6310e) they found when the phone was switched on and off by a remote computer Delta waves were reduced for close to an hour after the phone was shut off. The test subjects, who were sleep deprived the night before, were not aware of when the phones were switched off and could not fall asleep for nearly an hour. The significance of the study is that electromagnetic radiation does have an effect on mental behavior when it is transmitted at a certain frequency (Fields, 2008).

Alpha (8-13 Hz)

Our Alpha waves take over when we are alert, yet relaxed. We are awake but resting (Neurohealth, 2020). "The Alpha wave regulates the shift of attention between external and internal inputs." (Fields, 2008).

Rodney Croft, of the Brain Science Institute, Swinburne University of Technology in Melbourne, Australia, conducted a study using a Nokia 6110 cell phone. In a double-blind experiment it was revealed that when the phone was transmitting, Alpha wave patterns were increased. The greatest increase was in brain tissue directly beneath the cell phone (Fields, 2008).

Beta (14-30 Hz)

Beta waves represent rapid activity. Generally, it is regarded as the normal and dominant rhythm in an alert or anxious person It is the state the brain is in when our eyes are open, and we are listening and thinking. Beta waves are present during problem solving, decision making, and processing information. There are three Beta bands, low, midrange and high (NTD, 2019).

One study revealed that cell phone usage increased the level of beta waves. This increase lead to stress, anxiety, physical and mental discomforts, including muscular pain (Nandan, 2014).

Gamma (above 30 Hz)

Gamma waves are associated with our behaviors, feelings, thinking, integrated thoughts and high-level information processing. Gamma waves are the only frequency group that are in found in every part of the brain. Gamma waves are highly linked with our vision. A good memory is associated with 40Hz activity and a deficiency in 40Hz activity is associated with learning disabilities (NTD, 2019).

There are many reports of "voice to skull" This is what is also known as the "God Voice". These frequencies are used to put voices in people's heads. There is a Ted talk by Woody Norris where he explains his inventions and how LRAD is used. It is titled "Hypersonic Sound and Other Inventions" (Miller, 2003)

CHAPTER 4.

OUR BODIES SPEAK IN FREQUENCIES

Since our bodies speak in frequencies it is very important to understand how all electromagnetic fields including **5G**, might affect them.

Our bodies frequencies and vibrations have been discovered by using a highly sensitive laser device. They discovered that the vibrations are related to the cardiovascular system. This system has its own system, which has its own appropriate movements occurring simultaneously with the work of the heart. The first was a wave connected with the heartbeat, the second is the respiratory rhythm and the third is intwined with emotional tension (Traube-Heringwaves). Consequently, it could be possible to judge the human emotional state via the amplitude.

frequency response of these waves. (National Research Nuclear University, 2016).

The average frequency of the human body during daytime is 62 to 68 Hz. According to Tainio, of Tainio Technology, the body resonates frequency between 62 to 72 Hz when healthy . As the frequency drops due to environmental and physiological factors, (which includes our current electric magnetic fields and 5G) our immune system is compromised, and disease is more apt to develop.

Many pollutants have been found to lower healthy body frequency. Processed or canned foods, for example, tend to have a frequency of zero. On the contrary, fresh produce has up to 15 MHz, dried herbs from 12 to 22 MHz and fresh herbs from 2 MHz. Royal Rife used frequencies to heal the body, and Nicola Tesla suggested the elimination of certain outside frequencies that interfere with our bodies to resist disease. Tesla discovered the following frequencies regarding the body, disease and foods:

THE HEALTHY BODY

Genius Brain Frequency 80–82 MHz
Brain Frequency Range 72–90 MHz
Normal Brain Frequency 72 MHz
Human Body 62–78 MHz
Human Body from Neck up 72–78 MHz
Human Body from Neck down 60–68 MHz
Thyroid and Parathyroid glands 62–68 MHz
Thymus gland 65–68 MHz
Heart is 67–70 MHz
Lungs 58–65 MHz
Liver 55–60 MHz
Pancreas 60–80 MHz
THE DISEASED BODY
Colds and the Flu start at 57–60 MHz
Disease starts at 58 MHz
Candida overgrowth starts at 55 MHz

Receptive to Epstein Barr at 52 MHz
Receptive to Cancer at 42 MHz
Death begins at 25 MHz
FOODS
Fresh Foods 20–27 Hz
Fresh Herbs 20–27 Hz
Dried Foods 15–22 Hz
Dried Herbs 15–22 Hz
Processed/Canned Food Zero Hz0 to
27 Hz. (Schomburg, 2014)
5G at 60 hz
At 60Ghz , 5G resonates with the
oxygen molecule and gives oxygen a
reverse polarity that makes it less
usable to the human body. That means
at high concentrations we humans can
suffocate at street level. At lower
concentrations flu like symptoms can
occur.

**HIGHER FREQUENCY MEANS
BETTER HEALTH**

Higher frequency **in** the body, results
in better health. That does not mean
high frequency waves from **outside**

the body results in better health. According to Dr. Valerie Hunt, each toxic substance distorts the negative equilibrium that exists in the cellular level. Toxins depolarize the cell, which then becomes south polarized and ends up losing its ability to attract magnetic energy. This can lead to physical, psychological, emotional, and spiritual diseases.

It has been shown that a normal healthy body has a frequency of 62–72 MHz. When the body drops below this frequency, we begin to get into illness and disease states. For example, if our frequency drops to 58 MHz, then we are likely to get a cold or flu. If our frequency drops to 42 MHz, we become susceptible to cancer within the body. The lower the frequency, the closer we are to death.

CHAPTER 5.

SMART METERS

Smart meters are digital meters that are replacing older analog meters at residential and commercial buildings. A smart meter can measure data regarding electricity use and peak demand. They communicate to the power company wirelessly and eliminate the necessity of sending a person out to read the meter. As with **5G** technology there are those that state the meters are not harmful and those who say they are. For the sake of safety will want to talk about what might happen if the smart meter is unhealthy.

DIRTY ELECTRICITY

Smart meters might cause "dirty electricity" . All of us who have electricity in our homes, have an electrical current that flows continually through the wiring in our walls. As the electrical current travels, it creates an electromagnetic field that radiates outward at a ninety-degree angle. The radiation reaches out of the wall into the room. When there is a spike in the electricity it creates what is known as an EMI (Electromagnetic Interference). The EMI is what is called "Dirty Electricity".

Each Smart Meter is equipped with a radio frequency transmitter. The transmitter is used to transmit wireless microwave radiation. That is what enables the meter to connect to the Smart Grid where it wirelessly submits data to the utility company. There is also a "Switching Mode Power Supply" (SMPS) that is responsible for 'stepping down' the 240 V alternating current (AC) coming in from the utility pole power lines to the 2-10 V of direct current (DC) that is required to run the Smart Meter's own digital electronics. These digital electronics are responsible for recording your energy usage. Each **millisecond** the SMPS emits sharp spikes of electrical bursts. This takes place 24/7. Along with the RF radiation emitted from the transmitter, the constant pulsing of high frequencies causes constant EMI or "Dirty Electricity" in the building or home that the Smart Meter is attached to. The dirty electricity harms the biological systems of people, animals and plants that encounter its field (Body Health, 2020).

Common Symptoms Caused by Smart Meter Radiation and Dirty Electricity

Following are some of the symptoms reported:

Stress and Irritability – Including mood swings. Some individuals report that their mood changes from room to room. Backed by studies published in the *Journal of Chemical Neuroanotomy*

Skin Problems – Rashes and facial flushing.

Arthritis and Body Pain - Stiff joints from excess inflammation, damage to the nervous system causing body pain.

Trouble Sleeping – Sleep quality and duration is disrupted. A published article *"Effect of A nighttime Magnetic Field Exposure on Sleep Patterns in young Women"* revealed night-time exposure to EMI and EMF radiation is more damaging that day-time exposure.

Heart Problems – An expert on magnetic field therapy, Dr. Pawluk, states EMF radiation easily reach human and animal tissues. That includes heart tissues. There are many heart problems associated with EMI and EMF radiation including:
- Cardiac arrhythmia
- Bradycardia

- Tachycardia
- Premature Ventricular Contractions
- Premature Atrial Contractions
- Atrial Fibrillation or Atrial Flutter

Eye Problems – Burning or painful eyes, reduced visual acuity, floaters, pressure within or behind the eyes, cataracts.

Seizures – Those with epileptic seizures could have more acute negative reactions.

Other symptoms include:
- Headaches
- Vertigo
- Fatigue
- Tinnitus
- Sinus Problems
- Vertigo
- Nausea
- Leg Cramps
- Respiratory Problems

72

Endocrine and Thyroid Disorders

Prevention Regarding Smart Meters

In the case of the Smart Meter you can buy a radiofrequency (RF) meter to measure the amount of radiation emitting from it and the dirty electricity in your home or building. You can also buy a Faraday Cage to cover it. The radiation from the Smart Meter goes out 40ft, the Faraday Cage blocks 98% of it. There are instructions on the internet about how to build your own Faraday cage for about $10.00

Dirty electricity can be blocked using devices such as Greenwave dirty electricity filters. The device plugs into power strips and outlets to reduce dirty electricity.
More prevention information is provided in the following chapters.

CHAPTER 6.

5G TECHNOLOGIES

5G is not all about fast WIFI and better cell phone calls. Following are some of the technologies that use or will be using 5G.

Driverless Cars

Self-driving cars use several technologies including cameras, ultrasound, radio antennas and radar. The cars on the road today use these technologies in conjunction with one another. In example, Tesla's driverless car technology, Autopilot, uses 360-degree cameras for visibility, and front facing radar for analyzation of surroundings. What makes the car more reliable is the implantation of 5G cellular networks. 5G networks will allow seamless communication from one vehicle to another. Also, IoT (a piece of hardware with a sensor that

74

transmits data from one place to another over the Internet) will coordinate traffic lights, etc. Self-driving cars will require extremely low latency. For that reason, the goal of 5G is to achieve latencies below the 1-millisecond mark. Mobile devices will be able to send and receive information in less than one-thousandth of a second, appearing instantaneous to the user

Smart Devices

A **few** examples of smart devices"

- Refrigerators
- Watches
- Fire alarms
- Door locks
- Bicycles
- Medical sensors
- Fitness Trackers
- Smart security systems
- Televisions

Virtual Reality

In virtual reality a computer technology is used to create a three-dimensional simulated world. The user can explore and manipulate as if it were real. There are dozens of devices already on the market. Opinions differ about what is actually a true virtual reality experience but here are some general uses:

Three-dimensional images that appear to the user as life sized.

The ability to read the user's motions, especially the eyes and head to adjust the images to correspond with the users change of perspective.

CHAPTER 7

TAKE PREVENTATIVE ACTION

Everything we have been researching points at **5G** as well as all WIFI waves, deplete our oxygen levels. Now is the time to take measures to improve our blood oxygen. According to J.E. Ante 5G at 60Ghz resonates with the oxygen molecule and gives oxygen a reverse polarity that makes it much less usable to the human body. At high concentrations of 5G usage you get suffocation of humans at street level. And at lower doses you get flu like symptoms which are the exact same symptoms as the flu with this lowered oxygen uptake by the body.

It is a good idea to monitor blood oxygen level. The best way is by an arterial blood gas or ABG test. This test requires a blood sample from an artery, usually the right side. It is very accurate but can be painful and expensive.

We suggest buying a pulse oximeter. It is a small device that can be used at home or when traveling. It is a small clip that is put on a finger, ear or toe that measures blood oxygen indirectly by light absorption through a person's pulse. Although it is not as accurate as the ABG test, because it can be influence by factors such as nail polish, dirty fingers, bright lights, and poor circulation to the extremities, it is quick, easy and not painful. A pulse oximeter can be found online and at most medical supply stores at a modest cost (Silva, 2020).

Normal and Low Blood Oxygen Levels

Using the **ABG test**, the normal level for blood oxygen is between 75 and 100 millimeters of mercury (mm Hg). If the level goes below 60 it is considered low and may require oxygen supplementation. Each case depends upon the individual and their doctor's advice.

When the level is below 60 it can lead to hypoxemia, a condition that causes the body to have a difficult time delivering oxygen to all of its' tissues, cells and organs (Silva, 2020).

Normal oxygen saturation levels as measured by **pulse oximetry** range from 95% to 100%. Values under 90% are considered low.

Does that mean you should panic if you have an oxygen level 89? Not necessarily. First you need to understand which level you are talking about: Your blood oxygen level or your oxygen saturation. If you have a blood oxygen level between 100 mm Hg and 75 mm Hg, you are doing quite well! So that means that if this is the oxygen level you are speaking about, oxygen level 89, oxygen level 86 and oxygen level 80 would all be just fine. However, if you were actually talking about your oxygen saturation, (measured by a pulse oximeter) a normal oxygen saturation level should fall between 95% and 100%; in this case, a measurement of 89% would be worrisome.

Keep in mind an oxygen level below 88% (using the pulse oximeter) for any period of time is dangerous and warrants a trip to the hospital.

How to Increase Our Oxygen Level

First and foremost, **STOP SMOKING!** We understand that this will not be easy. If we want to avoid being sick, it is our responsibility to break bad habits that deplete our body of oxygen. Do whatever it takes to avoid smoking. Whenever possible, we should open our windows Fresh air is essential for breathing. We must be careful, though, to keep on eye on our local air quality. We should not open our windows up to smoky air or smog. Those living in an area where this is the norm, should consider an indoor air filtration system or other items that purify home air. Keep in mind to carefully choose electronic air purifiers because many of them can produce lung irritants.

Avoid breathing smoke from campfires and fireplaces.

Avoid breathing chemicals from cleaning products, paints etc. Artists should be aware of toxic chemicals and heavy metals in the paints they use.

Growing plants inside our home can increase oxygen. Ferns work great for this purpose because they are easy to grow, maintain and do not need much sun.

Exercise is another way to increase oxygen. We should check with our doctor about what type and amount of exercise is best for us to do each day. As our breathing rate increases our lungs absorb more oxygen.

Prayer and meditation daily reduce stress. Our beginning routine should emphasize deep breathing. Five to ten minutes a day of relaxed and focused breathing will help tremendously.

Fresh foods rich in iron are also helpful. There are foods that can aid in improving our blood oxygen levels Eat foods such as small amounts of organic red meat, poultry, fish legumes and green leafy vegetables. The reason to focus on iron rich foods, is to be certain we do not have an iron deficiency. Iron deficiency decreases our body's ability to process oxygen and can make us feel sick and tired (Lung Institute, 2016).

Drink plenty of water to oxygenate and expel carbon dioxide. Our lungs need to be hydrated and drinking enough water will influences our oxygen levels. Drink from glass not plastic bottles. Be aware of water sold in plastic because the plastic can leach toxins into the water. Keep in mind too much water can throw off electrolytes.

To oxygenate and expel carbon dioxide, our lungs need to be hydrated. Therefore, drinking enough water influences oxygen levels.

Be careful about aromas and fragrances that contain oxygen stealing chemicals Best to burn all-natural beeswax candles. Also, do not use lead wicks.

Consider a low salt sodium diet. Cutting out the salt can lead to increased oxygenation via the kidney and the blood.

Breathing Exercises

Diaphragmatic Breathing

Many of us do not know that there is a right way to breathe. Individuals with limited lung capacity often fall into the habit of taking short, shallow breaths into their chest. If a person's chest rises as they take a breath, it is a likely indicator of improper breathing. A proper breath will draw air into the lungs, pushing the diaphragm down and visibly expanding the belly. Follow these steps to engage in deep, diaphragmatic breathing:

1. Sit up straight, with one hand on the stomach and the other on the chest.
2. Inhale slowly and deeply through the nostrils, feeling the stomach expand with each full, diaphragmatic breath.
3. Exhale slowly out of the mouth.

84

4. Repeat six or more times each minute for up to 15 minutes.

The 4-7-8 Technique

The 4-7-8 breathing technique not only increases oxygen, it can help a person fall asleep quickly because of the 4-7-8 technique's ability to ease tension and promote relaxation. Performing the following focused breathing exercise twice a day will help minimize food cravings, reduce anxiety and provide relief from insomnia.

Breathe out fully through the mouth, creating a wind-like "whoosh" noise.

Keeping the mouth closed, inhale through the nose and silently count to four.

Hold this breath while counting to seven.

Exhale through the mouth for a count of eight, repeating the "whoosh" sound.

Repeat steps two through four daily five times.

85

Buteyko Nose Breathing

Invented in the 1950's a Russian scientist invented Buteyko breathing to aid asthmatic patients and others with respiratory problems. As often happens, the medical field scoffed at a breathing technique to ease symptoms without the use of medications. Many people have used this technique and find it a natural and effective way to get relief from asthma sleep apnea and hypertension. The method balances the body's oxygen and carbon dioxide levels. It is best to make it part of your daily routine. Initially, seniors should perform the exercise under supervision to avoid hyperventilation caused by improper technique.

In a quiet, comfortable place, sit up straight and focus on breathing.

Keeping the mouth closed, inhale slowly through the nostrils to fill the lungs.

Exhale through the nostrils, slowly expelling air from the lungs ,until you feel compelled to inhale.
Repeat steps two and three five time (Shinde, 2020)

Foods to Oxygenate Cells

A diet high in oxygen is filled with raw foods consisting of fruits, green vegetables and sprouted seeds. As we have already suggested foods rich in iron are also helpful, such as, Farm raised meat, poultry, fish from lakes, streams and the ocean, legumes and green leafy vegetables.

Leavy green vegetables also contain chlorophyll which is close in atomic structure to human blood. Eating green vegetables allows the chlorophyll to aid the blood to transport oxygen to our cells. Chlorophyll rich foods include broccoli, kale, spinach, mustard greens, spirulina chlorella and blue-green algae.

Fruits, vegetables, legumes and whole grains are complex carbohydrates which can also help the blood transport oxygen to cells.

Juices from fruits and vegetables also put antioxidants into the bloodstream to aid in oxygen uptake. Antioxidants support efficient oxygen use (Rejuvinea Health, 2014).

Tinnitus

Both **5g** and the WIFI we have in place now, can cause tinnitus especially through the cell phone. A report that appeared in the *British Medical Journal* reported that extended cell phone use is a cause of tinnitus. The report states that 10-15% of people using cellphones experience some degree of tinnitus. The number is growing as more individuals are using cell phones more often and for longer periods of time. The study excluded those with obvious tinnitus triggers such as ear disease or noise-induced hearing loss.

It was discovered that most of the tinnitus was one-sided. Many the test subjects reported the ringing and living with sounds that aren't really there was "distressing and lowered the quality of life".

The researchers suggested there is a potential link between mobile phones and tinnitus as the cochlea and the auditory pathway directly absorb energy emitted by the cell phone. That means the wireless connectivity required for cell phone use damages our hearing mechanism.

There is no known cure for the ringing but there are some to treat the symptoms.

The very best treatment is to avoid the problem in the first place. Avoid turning earbuds up to a loud volume. Give your ears a break by using the speakerphone. It also a good idea to keep calls as short as possible.

Supplements

See your doctor or nutritionist to determine the correct amount for you.

Antioxidants such as Vitamins A, C (with bioflavonoids) E and selenium are strong antioxidants.

B-Vitamins aid in the synthetization of a protein that carries oxygen in the blood.

Vitamin D3 helps with oxygen uptake in the blood.

NOTE: If you have sudden problems breathing, leave the area or building you are in to see if it improves your symptoms.

Massage

Massage therapy is the use of rubbing, kneading and working muscles and soft tissues in order to bring about healing to the body.

When your body is massaged, circulation improves, and oxygen and other nutrients are brought to the body tissues.

Massage can relieve muscle tension and pain, increase flexibility and mobility, clear lactic acid and other waste and enhance immune function.

The types of massage therapy are Swedish, sports massage, neuromuscular (deep tissue), reflexology and cranial sacral.

Reducing Exposure

We realize that most people are not going to throw away their devices or even turn them off. Yet, there are some steps that can be taken to reduce exposure to EMF waves including 5G.

- **Unplug your Wi-Fi router** at night or when not in use.
- **Use ethernet cords.** Ethernet cords also help stop hackers that can easily get into your wireless network.
- **When not using your devices, turn them off** or keep them in airplane mode.
- **Unplug your smart** tv when not in use. As a matter of fact, avoid them altogether.
- As we spoke about in the section regarding smart meters, **clean your home of dirty electricity.**
- **Separate devices such as tablets and cells phones from your body** when not in use. When possible use speakerphone during phone calls to keep the phone away from your ear.
- **Replace Wireless with Wired Devices** Some devices — such as your wireless keyboard,

headset, and mouse — function only when they are transmitting a wireless signal. Replace these devices with a wired version.

- **Keep wireless devices out of the bedroom**, including digital alarm clocks.
- **Do not use Bluetooth earbuds**

CELLPHONE AND TABLET

To protect ourselves from the harmful effects of cellphones, we use EMF shields. These devices come in several sizes and you can stick them on your phone and tablets. Some work through quantum physics. Please be careful when choosing. One way to make certain they work is to purchase an EMF meter to measure before and after installation. It is good to measure the levels of radiation within 100 feet of your home. Research all the consumer products in this category so that you can protect yourself as much as possible.

Buy an EMF Protection Cell Phone Case. Cell phones have become indispensable for so many of us. They give us freedom while keeping us connected to work, home, family and the world. But, every time you hold your cell phone to your ear, you are absorbing over 50% of the cell phone radiation it transmits. There are many radiation protection cell phone cases available on the internet.

As mentioned previously try not to have bodily contact with your phone, tablet or laptop. Most cell phone manufacturers recommend keeping at least 10mm of space between you and your phone. Avoid putting your phone in your pocket or your sports bra! And don't sleep with your cell phone next to your bed. If you must keep your phone next to you at night – for example, if you use the alarm feature on your phone – be sure to keep it at least six feet away. Women **DO NOT** put your laptop on your lap if you are trying to get pregnant. Men do not put the laptop on your lap because it lowers sperm count.

Take some time away from your electronics. Abstain from using your cell phone for long periods of time, **including never keeping your cell phone in your bedroom**. If possible, keep your mobile devices five to ten feet away from you. When traveling with your cell phone, store it in an EMF protective bag.

All computers, tablets, cell phones should have a **blue light protector**. To avoid macular degeneration. You can find these on Amazon or Ebay.

Crystals and Stones

Crystals and stones can help block, absorb, or change the EMF waves.

Organite

Orgonite, which reportedly scatters electromagnetic fields and turns them into beneficial ones. (Wagner, 2020). Orgonite is a composite developed by the late Dr. Wilhelm Reich. This composite can change harmful electromagnetic fields and transform them into harmless beneficial fields. It accomplishes this by emitting negative ions into the environment. You can place orgonite on your body, around your home, office and garden to protect you.

Elite Shungite is an equally powerful, EMF resistant stone. Shungite attenuates electromagnetic emissions from electrical grids, computers, cell-phones, Wi-Fi, appliances, and other electronic devices—this means shungite transforms harmful manmade EMFs into wave forms that are more compatible with our biology." It can purify water. This is all due to the crystal's carbon content. Shungite is the only known natural mineral to contain fullerenes, a crystalline form of carbon. Fullerenes is an antioxidant that neutralizes free radicals. Fullerenes are anti-everything harmful to us including viruses, bacteria, fungus, pathogens, and all those harmful chemicals we are exposed to daily like fluoride and chlorine in our drinking water. Shungite is an ancient stone, believed to be almost 2 billion years old. Shungite was formed when there were no life forms on earth, deep within the earth's crust. The main deposit of Shungite on earth comes from the Zazhoginskoye deposit near Lake Onega in the Shunga region of Karelia, North West of Russia.

Shungite paint is a great material for wall coating. The color is magnetic deep black so black color would have to be part of your homes color scheme. To create shungite paint; mix shungite powder with water at approximately a 1:2 ratio. The resulting mixture will be creamy in texture. You can then use it as a paste or paint that becomes solid when dry. Make certain to keep stirred so that it is uniform without clots or other irregularities.

 After making shungite paste/paint, distribute it evenly on the surface you wish to paint and let it dry. The results depend on your abilities as a repairman and your artistic interests. Use different strokes to create magnificent patterns of shungite paint on your walls. In order to achieve the color and the consistency you need apply several layers of shungite paste after the previous layer is completely dry. If you have trouble with shungite paste staying in solid form on the wall you can mix it with regular wall paint, but again make sure that it is mixed evenly.

 Shungite paint can also be used for decorating smaller pieces of interior and it is also a conductive paint, so it can be used in that way. The evenly spread paint will ensure comprehensive protection of your household for years to come.

Be careful where you live. Avoid living near a cell tower, power station, or **5G** antenna pole (Wagner, 2020)

We have chosen to wear Q3 **Photonic Holographic Frequency** bands. The bands harmonize the body's frequencies in order for cells to naturally protect and heal.

Aluminum

We are not suggesting that you and your family make hats out of aluminum foil. But aluminum foil does shield or block radio waves. As a matter of fact, the aluminum hats sold on the internet can cause more problems because the waves expand from the head into the body.

Does Aluminum Foil Protect Against Radio Frequency Radiation?

Aluminum foil does block, or shield, radio frequency waves. Since aluminum conducts electricity it forms a barrier against the waves. Faraday Cages, as mentioned in the smart meter section of this book, use aluminum mesh to block radiation. Take a look at your microwave and you will see metal mesh layered in the window this is much like the Faraday cage material.

It is important to know that the aluminum does not absorb the EMF it just blocks it. The aluminum needs to be between you and the EMF producing device (Wi-Fi router, cell phones, etc.), or your cells may still be affected by EMF radiation. You can store your home electronics in an aluminum foil lined box. This uses the same principles as the Faraday cage to block EMF radiation.

The thicker the better. Aluminum sheeting can be purchased in rolls at hardware stores.

Earthing

Our bodies are conductive and contain a large amount of charged ions. These ions are called electrolytes and live in our blood and around our cells. When the electrons in our body come into close contact of AC voltage and EMF radiation they wiggle. That's why our body AC voltage (as measured with a multimeter) goes up when we get closer to an appliance or AC electrical wiring. When our body is grounded the electrons cannot wiggle. Earthing can protect us from some electromagnetic fields, especially from low-frequency EMFs. When we are in direct contact with the surface of the Earth, negatively charged ions transfer into our bodies, which can help neutralize the positively charged oxidants. This can help reduce inflammation and improve our overall feeling of wellness. This energy transfer by direct contact with the Earth's surface is appropriately called **"Earthing,"** or more commonly known as **"Grounding"**.

Gaetan Chevalier PHD and James L. Oschman PHD have published an article *Understanding Earthing (Grounding)* on the topic of how earthing can protect our bodies from EMF waves. They state, "earthing is an overlooked factor in public health" and that it is "a missing link with broad and significant implications" for health.

Earthing is most effective at deflecting low EMF's of 100,000 Hz and less. That means it can protect you from EMFs emitted from AC electrical wiring and most household appliances. No research has been conducted on earthing regarding high frequencies such as wi-fi and smart meters. Although it is unclear if earthing offers any protection, it is clear the healthier a person is, the more likely they are to withstand 5G and earthing protects our health (Better Earthing, 2020).

How to Ground or Earth

The earth contains antioxidants that allow our bodies to achieve equilibrium at the cellular level. All a person needs to do to allow the earth to aid in our health is walk barefoot or sit in the dirt, grass, sand or even on concrete. Since these surfaces are conductive and allow the Earth's energy to flow through them into our bodies.

Water is also conductive so swimming or standing in water is ideal for grounding.

If you do not like to get wet or dirty, the best conductive footwear are shoes with thin leather soles. You can also purchase grounding socks that contain conductive materials so you can ground without physically touching the dirt.

Keep in mind that there are places where the ground is not good for our wellbeing, such as places with and abundance of EMF waves like crowded cities or manufacturing facilities, near cell towers or anywhere high-tech equipment sends electricity into the soil to the ground. In this type of ground the current (normally safe and healthy) varies and excess ground current can cause harm. When finding your outdoor grounding place, make certain it is away from technology and toxins.

If you are confined indoor there are many tools that can be purchased that can connect you to the earth's frequencies without going outside. Grounding devices used in the home or

103

office connect us to the Earth's electrons via a grounded wall outlet. There is controversy about whether these devises benefit people. Some people say the equipment allows them to feel better, but others say they feel worse. Those feeling worse might be in a high EMF environment such as an office or apartment building with an abundance of technology. The ambient EMF might be using their bodies as a pathway to the ground. Therefore, the body could be attracting the EMF in the room before it is grounded by flowing through the person to the mat. Using a grounded wall outlet does not use electricity, but it may pick up a stray current in the home's circuitry (DeBaun, 2020).

Sound Therapy

As we pointed out in chapter 4, our bodies speak in frequencies. It is the language all life understands at a cellular level. It is the foundation upon which every physiological process is based. It is the critical means of communication between all things on a macrocosmic as well as microcosmic level. Our cells exchange information and regulate body functions through the sending and receiving of specific frequencies. This cell signaling precedes and regulates all biochemical actions.

Our bodies natural frequency signals can become scrambled by harmful electromagnetic fields such as 5G. When this scrambling occurs, our body loses its' ability to self-regulate and maintain healthy organ functions.

The electromagnetic energy generated by and surrounding our body – has always been kept in balance by the larger enveloping electromagnetic field generated by the earth, the atmosphere, and the ecosphere. When our frequency became disrupted, it could usually right itself in a few days or weeks because we were surrounded by a powerful natural energy field emitted by nature. We would automatically entrain with that field and come back into balance.

Because of WIFI, **5g,** and increasing radioactivity in our environment our natural healing harmonics have become weakened. Our environment is so toxic from unnatural chaotic frequencies, such as WIFI and **5G,** it is nearly impossible to maintain a healthy balance. This is where sound frequency therapy comes in.

When unhealthy frequencies such as WIFI signals disrupt cellular function and alter the cell's vibration to such an extent that its ability to send, receive, and accurately interpret signals is compromised, then the introduction of the appropriate healthy frequency will restore that cell to balance through the properties of resonance.

"Resonance is a phenomenon in which a vibrating system or external force drives another system to oscillate with greater amplitude at a specific preferential frequency."

106

Sound is an efficient frequency carrier, even more so than light. That is because our bodies are about 75% fluid and sounds travel father in water than in light (Whitehawk, 2018).

Rife Machine

A good sound therapy instrument, although not FDA approved, is a rife frequency machine that uses both sound and light frequencies. With this type of machine, you get the best of both worlds. You can search the internet to find the best one available. Such a machine also has an attachment that allows the user to make energized water. Energized water is charged with a specific frequency that helps strengthen our DNA strands.

Tuning Forks

Tuning forks emit vibrational sound waves. Traditionally they are used to tune musical instruments. Tuning Fork Therapy is a gentle, non-invasive acoustic therapy. This sound and vibrational therapy uses solfeggio tuning to help balance the energy of your body. Solfeggio tuning is a vibrational frequency that aids in moving energy, removing energy blocks, and increasing energy flow. As a result, Tuning Fork Therapy may help reduce pain, increase circulation, balance emotions, and increase overall energy.

The vibration of a tuning fork is felt as it resonates through muscle, bones, and organs creating entrainment. This is synchronization of the body's systems, organs, and tissues to the frequency of the fork reaching a harmonic natural rhythm. The treatment stimulates healing of tissue at the cellular level getting to the root cause of disharmony.

It works because each of our tissues, organs and cells have their own frequency. Musical instruments have varying sound waves, which penetrate the human body, causing vibrations within the cell. Specific vibrations strengthen healthy cells while regenerating weaker cells.

Tuning forks used for sound healing come in a variety of sets and frequencies. By directing the sound waves of correct tuning forks at key acupuncture and reflexology points, the sound travels through the body to the appropriate organ, gland, bone, or tissue. The healing frequency directs the body's cells to tune up to their proper healthy pitch enabling them to function as they should. For those sensitive to electro-magnetic frequency and radiation (EMFs and EMRs), tuning forks provide an alternative and effective solution.

Bracelets, Necklaces, Other Jewelry and Clothing

There is a wide assortment of bracelets, necklaces, other jewelry and necklaces that claim to protect us from 5G frequencies. The only way to know for certain if they work, is to do a before and after test with an EMF meter. We have purchased these devices and most past the test. We advise everyone to be prudent when purchasing these products.

CHAPTER 8.

TIPS FOR A HEALTHY IMMUNE SYSTEM

It is of utmost importance to boost our immune systems in order to withstand any health crisis that may occur. If the **5G** rollout doe indeed cause immune challenges, healthy people are going to have the best chance of survival.

Following are some ways to improve your immune system.

ESSENTIAL OILS

- Oregano
- Thyme
- Cinnamon
- Hyssop
- Thieves
- Orange Oil

These oils have been known to boost the immune system and are strong virus fighters. Keep in mind that they

111

are very powerful, and it is best to talk to a practitioner who can recommend the correct one's for you and your family.

HERBAL MEDICINES AND SUPPLEMENTS

KEEP IN MIND SOME SUPPLEMENTS CAN BE TOXIC AT HIGH LEVELS. SEE YOUR HEALTH CARE PROVIDER BEFORE TAKING SUPPLEMENTS

Herbal medicine, also called botanical medicine or phytomedicine, refers to the practice of using a plant's seeds, berries, roots, leaves, bark or flowers for medicinal purposes.

Although most herbalists agree that medication is best in emergency situations, they view herbal medicines as **the way for a patient to resist disease**, as well as provide nutritional and **immunological support**. The goal of herbal medication is both prevention and cure.

112

Some top supplements to a heathy strong immune system:

- **Colloidal Silver** is antibacterial, anti-microbial, anti-viral and anti-inflammatory (see your health professional because some people have sensitivities to silver)
- **Zinc**- promotes healthy cell and healing ability
- **B6**- supports blood cells and the nervous system
- **Vitamin C**- powerful antioxidant that fights free radicals
- **Vitamin E**- powerful antioxidant that helps fight infections
- **Elderberry**- boosting immunity. It can protect against infections and bacteria. * It is contraindicated in children with diabetes or

anyone with an autoimmune disorder

- **Glutathione** – along with other amazing benefits it supports a strong immune system

HOMEOPATHIC MEDICINE

Homeopathy is an alternative medicine that treats a wide range of health conditions through a practice called the "law of similars." This principle states that a substance that can cause disease in an individual can cure that disease if given in small doses known as homeopathic dilutions.

Homeopathic preparations, called remedies, must be prepared in a certain way, and the dilution used will depend on the symptoms being treated. *(YODER, 2017)*

- **Virex** is a homeopathy from Nutriwest is a great product for fighting viruses
- **Total Bac-T** also from Nutriwest fights bacteria

INTESTINAL TRACT

Keep in mind that most of our immune cells are developed in the intestinal tract. A good bowel cleanse will help your immune system. Eating a cup of sauerkraut daily (read the label to avoid high fructose corn syrup etc). will also help keep your intestines in balance. Eat plenty of fresh fruits and vegetables and stay away from refined sugar. Exercise, stress reduction and plenty of rest all aid in keeping our intestinal tract healthy. Avoid deep fried foods, white sugar, white flour and food high in saturated fats because they can destroy the immune system.

DETOXING

To keep a healthy immune system, we must get rid of the toxins in our bodies. Following are some ideas to rid our bodies of toxins.

Infrared Saunas:

Far infrared saunas (FIR) provides many of the health benefits of natural sunlight without any of the dangerous effects of solar radiation. Traditional steam saunas raise the temperature of the air to a very high level within the chamber to warm the body. Some people have difficulty breathing in this extremely warm air. FIR saunas work differently Instead of heating the air within the enclosure, FIR saunas heat the body directly. The result is a lower power bill and deeper tissue penetration. In the FIR sauna, the body perspires and receives all the healthy benefits but avoids the harmful and extremely hot air of a traditional steam sauna. FIR saunas are safe for all ages.

Some people do not perspire for the first 4 to 6 sessions, it is as though their body has to be trained to sweat.

Benefits from Infrared Saunas include:

Better circulation and increased energy: The saunas emit FIR energy that is absorbed by human cells, causing a physical phenomenon called "resonance". Thus, the cellular activities are instantly invigorated, resulting in a better blood circulation and an overall improved metabolism.

Weight loss: FIR Sauna heat therapy can aid in weight loss by speeding up the metabolic process of vital organs and endocrine glans resulting in substantial caloric loss in a sauna heat session.

Cardiovascular health: The FIR sauna increases heart rate and blood circulation, crucial to maintaining one's health. The heart rate increases as more blood flow is diverted from the inner organs towards the extremities of the skin, without elevating blood pressure.

Detoxification: The skin is often referred to as the 3rd kidney, because it is believed to be responsible for elimination 30% of the body's waste. It can help eliminate chemicals and heavy metals from the body.

Stress Reduction and Relaxation: FIR Sauna heat treatment before a massage also helps prepare a client by creating an overall relaxing effect. It loosens the muscle tissue so the therapist can do a more thorough and effective massage.

Skin Beautification: FIR Sauna heat therapy allows increased blood circulation to carry great amounts of nutrients to the skin, thus promoting healthy tone and texture. It helps the skin to stay soft and eliminates dry skin.

Improved Immune System: A FIR heat treatment in the early stages of a cold or flu has been known to stop the disease before the symptoms occur.

The Infrared Sauna that we prefer, and use is from High Tech Health (800) 794-5355

Coffee Enemas:

Coffee enemas are powerful detoxifiers, due to some amazing compounds within the coffee that stimulate the liver to produce Glutathione S transferase, a chemical which is known to be the master detoxifier in our bodies. Glutathione S transferase binds to toxins and the toxins are then released out of the body along with the coffee.

Note organic coffee should be used not commercial coffee.

Reasons on why you should try a coffee enema:

- Reduces levels of toxicity by up to 600%

- Cleans and heals the colon, improving peristalsis.
- Increases energy levels, improves mental clarity and mood
- Helps with depression, bad moods, sluggishness
- Helps eliminate parasites and candida
- Improves digestion bile flow eases bloating
- Detoxifies the liver and helps repair the liver
- Can help heal chronic health conditions (along with eating a whole food diet)
- Helps ease "die off" or detox reactions during periods of fasting or juice fasting, cleansing, or healing
- Used regularly for healing in cancer patients

You can buy an enema kit online. Buy some premium ground ORGANIC coffee beans and keep them in the freezer until you need to use the coffee.

.Baths of Detoxification

Epsom Salts and Ginger: This bath opens pores and eliminates toxins and helps to eliminate pain. One cup Epsom salts and 2 tablespoons of ginger stirred in a cup of water first. Then added to bath is beneficial Do not remain in tub for more than 30 minutes.

Salt and Baking Soda: This bath counteracts the effects of radiation, whether from x-rays or cancer radiation treatments, fallout from the atmosphere or television radiation. Add one cup of baking soda and one to two cups ordinary coarse salt, Epsom salts or sea salt to a tub of water. You can soak for 20 minutes.

Apple Cider Vinegar bath: This is used when the body is too acidic. This is a quick way of restoring the acid-alkaline balance. Use one cup to 2 quarts of 100% organic apple cider vinegar to a bathtub of warm water.

Soak 40 to 45 minutes. This is excellent for excess uric acid in the body and is especially helpful for the joints and in conditions such as arthritis, bursitis, tendonitis, and gout.

Thymus Thump

The Thymus Thump can assist to neutralize negative energy, exude calm, revamp energy, support healing and vibrant health, and **boost your immune system.** It is simple but very effective energy technique involves tapping, thumping or scratching on the thymus point.

The thymus gland cannot be felt from the outside of the body. This is because it is located behind the sternum, also called the breastbone. You can thump in the middle of your chest with your fist (think Tarzan). Or, you may want to rub softly or firmly or scratch with four fingers of your hand. Do this for about 20 seconds and breathe deeply in and out.

Vitamin C

Platefuls of **vitamin C rich foods** like dark leafy greens, Brussels sprouts, kiwi fruit, broccoli, cantaloupe, cauliflower, kale, orange juice, red, green or yellow pepper, sweet potato, tomatoes and berries protect the thymus gland, a vital immune system organ.

CLEANSING

We also suggest that a person cleanses out toxins and parasites by doing a gut and liver cleanse once a year. There are many to choose from and your practitioner can guide you.

Also, heavy metals and fungus can be detoxed with the aid of supplements (Yoder, 2017).

Parasites

All our bodies are filled with parasitic organisms. When these parasites, as well as bacteria, and fungi are subjected to any WIFI including **5G** frequencies they can begin reproducing toxins in self-defense.

They also begin to reproduce rapidly to ensure their survival. This produces flu like symptoms. When parasites get killed off too quickly, we cannot drain them out of our system fast enough and can become toxic. We suggest doing gut cleanse now to get rid of toxins in a gentler manner.

CHAPTER 9.

STRESS

Stress is not good for our immune system. One way to relieve stress is to become educated about the problem at hand and work out a solution for dealing with it. Once you have accomplished that, take the steps needed to prepare and calm down. Worry is not a problems solver.

Constant worrying, negative thinking, and always expecting the worst can take a toll on your emotional and physical health.

There are steps you can take to turn off anxious thoughts. Chronic worrying is a mental habit that can be broken. You can train your brain to stay calm and look at life from a more balanced, less fearful perspective.

125

Create a daily "worry" period

Postponing worrying to a designated time can help relieve stress. Rather than trying to stop or get rid of an anxious thought, give yourself permission to have it, but put off dwelling on it until later. Create a "worry period." Choose a set time and place for worrying. It should be the same every day in example on the front porch from 4:00 pm to 4:15 pm. Make it early enough so you are not anxious right before bedtime. During your worry period, you're allowed to worry about whatever's on your mind. The rest of the day, however, is a worry-free zone. Write down your worries. If an anxious thought or worry comes into your head during the day, make a brief note of it and then continue about your day. Go over your "worry list" during the worry period. If the thoughts you wrote down are still bothering you, allow yourself to worry about them, but only for the time you've specified for your worry period.

126

As you examine your worries in this way, you'll often find it easier to develop a more balanced perspective. And if your worries don't seem important anymore, simply cut your worry period short and enjoy the rest of your day.

Meditation

Meditation is a wonderful practice that we urge all people to learn about and incorporate into their daily lives. Meditation is the practice of settling your mind through a conscious effort. The goal of meditation is for the mind to be quiet and free from stress using contemplation and reflection.

Some physical benefits of meditation include:

- A decrease in blood pressure and an improvement in breathing.

- A lower resting heart rate and lower stress chemicals such as cortisol.
- Reduces stress: Stress reduction is one of the most common reasons people try meditation
- Controls anxiety
- Promotes emotional health
- Enhances self-Awareness
- Lengthens attention span
- May reduce age-related memory loss
- Can generate kindness
- May help fight addiction

Taking small measures to reduce your anxiety can go a long way. There are many guided meditations that will help keep your mind focused

Basic mindfulness meditation

Find a quiet place

Sit on a comfortable chair or cushion, with your back straight, and your hands resting on the tops of your upper legs.

Close your eyes and breathe in through your nose, allowing the air downward into your lower belly. Let your abdomen expand fully.

Breathe out through your mouth.

Focus on an aspect of your breathing, such as the sensations of air flowing into your nostrils and out of your mouth, or your belly rising and falling as you inhale and exhale.

If your mind starts to wander, return your focus to your breathing with no judgment.

Try to meditate 3 or 4 times per week for 10 minutes per day. Every minute counts

EFT TECHNIQUE

Emotional Freedom Technique is a form of counseling intervention that draws on various theories of alternative medicine including acupuncture, neuro-linguistic programming, energy medicine and thought field therapy.

Yoga- a Hindu spiritual and ascetic discipline, a part of which, including breath control, simple meditation, and the adoption of specific bodily postures, is widely practiced for health and relaxation.

Tai chi- is an ancient Chinese tradition that, today ,is practiced as a graceful form of exercise, it involves a series of movements performed in a slow, focused manner and accompanied by deep breathing.

BREATHING--- Yoga includes various physical postures and breathing techniques, along with meditation.

Love yourself and your family. Love has a profound effect on our health. As the Bible teaches, "Love your neighbor as yourself".

NET Therapy

NET stands for Neuro Emotional Technique. It is a safe, effective and natural way to instantly resolve long-standing health problems that have an emotional or stressful component. People used to think emotions resided entirely in their brain. Now we know other parts of the body can hold emotions too. Have you ever experienced butterflies in your stomach before a speech, referred to something as a "pain in the neck" or felt a "lump in your throat". Clearly, emotions happen in our body, not just in our brain.

Most people say they would like to be healthy but something in their subconscious mind is not allowing this for them. So, before you can become healthy that Neuro Emotional connection needs to be cleared. We find where the block is within the body and release it. The body is amazing and can heal itself when given the proper tools (Yoder, 2017).

Louise Hay wrote a book called Heal Your Body in which she states that mental thought patterns form our experiences. She believes that every illness or condition we have relates to a specific emotion and that once you heal that emotional issue, your body can heal itself.

We have noted some of the most common conditions and their related emotional issues that have come into our office.

These include:

• Ankles- inflexibility and guilt, ankles represent the ability to receive pleasure.

• Bunions- lack of joy in meeting experiences in life.

• Elbow- represents changing directions and accepting new experiences.

- Wrist- represents movement and ease.

- Hips- Fear of going forward in major decisions, nothing to move forward to.

- Knees- stubborn pride and ego, inability to bend, fear, inflexibility, won't give in.

- Neck- refusing to see other sides of the question, stubbornness, inflexibility.

- Shoulders- represent our ability to carry our experiences in our life joyously, we make life a burden by our attitude.

- Spine- represents the support of life.

- Lower Spine- fear of money, lack of financial support.

- Middle Spine- guilt, stuck in all that mess back there, "get off my back".

- Upper Spine- lack of emotional support, feeling unloved, holding back love.

- Arthritis- feeling unloved, criticism, resentment.

- Bone breaks/fractures- repelling against authority.

- Bursitis- repressed anger.

- Inflammation- fear, seeing red, inflamed thinking.

- Joints- represents changes in direction in life and the ease of these movements.

- Loss of Balance- scattered thinking, not centered.

- Sciatica- being hypocritical, fear of money and/or the future.

- Slipped Disc -feeling totally unsupported by life, indecisive.

PRAYER

Prayer provides stress relief in a variety of ways. A prayer during these tense times relieves that feeling of loneliness. The belief that God is listening to our prayers and will help us is a source of hope to many individuals. With hope comes the strength to carry on.

Research shows that people who are more religious or spiritual use their spirituality to cope with life. Prayer can help us heal faster from illness and experience increased benefits of health and well-being. Spirituality enables us to stop trying to control things all by ourselves. It helps us feel part of a greater whole and understand that there is hope no matter what happens in life.

Make sure you have plenty of sleep every night. Relax and do not fear!

CHAPTER 10.

SUMMING IT UP

There are many theories regarding the dangers of **5g**. When a person goes looking, it is easy to find the advantages of the technology that 5g can push. To many 5g may seem like the least of our worries. After all, many people do not realize that the very reason they are "sick and tired", have immune challenges or other ailments can be caused by the WIFI system we have in place at this time.

It is our suggestion to protect yourself, you need to become educated and stay updated about 5g. Purchase an EMF meter and check your surroundings. Experiment with different EMF blocking recommendations and measure the difference.

We are not going to know anything for certain until that day we wake (if we wake up at all) to **5G**. If we are not prepared, we may be faced with an invisible enemy that we cannot recognize or fight.

BE PROACTIVE & STAY OUT OF FEAR. Remain positive and strong, and continue to improve your vibration through positive thinking, forgiveness, and with increased attention toward mental, emotional, and physical health.

OTHER BOOKS BY THE AUTHORS.

Thinking Outside the Box – A Chiropractor's View to Alternative Healthcare – Dr. Patricia L. Yoder , 2017

Unimaginable Reality – Protect Your Child from Child Pornography, Child Trafficking and Exposure to Internet Pornography – Barbara Schneider MS, 2017

The Five Major Stressors to Your Body! Discovering the Sources of Hidden Toxins – Patricia L. Yoder, D.C. and Barbara J. Schneider MS, 2019

Quarantined! How to Fearlessly Prepare for, Fight and Survive a Pandemic – Patricia L. Yoder DC and Barbara J. Schneider MS, 2020

WORKS CITED

EMFSA. (2020). *5G millimeter wave bandwith: US and China war-fighting domains (Space Command & Control)* . Retrieved from US ELECTROMAGNETIC DEFENSE TASK FORCE (EDTF).

Better Earthing. (2020). *Earthing and EMF / EMR Explained.* Retrieved from Better Earthing: https://betterearthing.com.au/earthing-and-emf-emr-explained/

Body Health. (2020, March 25). *Independent Lab Tests Show iPhone Exceeds FCC RF Safety Limits.* Retrieved from Safe Living: http://safeliving.tamers.biz/index.php/itemlist/user/716-superuser

Branswell, H. (2020, February 12). *Understanding pandemics: What they mean, don't mean, and what comes next with the coronavirus.* Retrieved from STAT: https://www.statnews.com/2020/02/12/understanding-pandemics-what-they-mean-coronavirus/

Brodkin, J. (2019, April 22). *Millimeter-wave 5G will never scale beyond dense urban areas, T-Mobile says.* Retrieved from ARSTECHNICA: https://arstechnica.com/informati on- technology/2019/04/millimeter-wave-5g-will-never-scale-beyond-dense-urban-areas-t-mobile-says/

CDC. (2020, February 14). *FAQS.* Retrieved from CDC: https://www.cdc.gov/coronavirus /2019-ncov/faq.html

DeBaun, D. (2020). *Does Grounding or Earthing Protect from EMF Radiation?* Retrieved from DefenderShield : https://www.defendershield.com/ does-grounding-or-earthing-protect-from-emf-radiation

Dinucci, M. (2019). *The Hidden Military Use of 5G Technology.*

Dovey, D. (2020, March 28). *RADIATION FROM CELLPHONES, WI-FI IS HURTING THE BIRDS AND THE BEES; 5G MAY MAKE IT WORSE.* Retrieved from Newsweek: https://www.newsweek.com/migr atory-birds-bee-navigation-5g-

technology-electromagnetic-
radiation-934830

etal, Z. (2009). Evaluation of the
Potential Biological Effects of
the60-GHz Millimeter Waves
Upon Human Cells. *IEEE
TRANSACTIONS ON
ANTENNAS AND
PROPAGATION.*

Fields, D. (2008, May 7). *Mind Control
by Cell Phone.* Retrieved from
NEUROLOGICAL HEALTH.

Freeman, M. (2020, January 5). *5G
Danger: 13 Reasons 5G Wireless
Technology Will Be a
Catastrophe for Humanity.*
Retrieved from Globol Research:
https://www.globalresearch.ca/5g
-danger-13-reasons-5g-wireless-
technology-will-be-a-
catastrophe-for-
humanity/5680503

Heinzman, A. (2019, July 23). *Not All
5G Is Equal: Millimeter Wave,
Low-Band, and Mid-Band
Explained.* Retrieved from How
To Geek:
https://www.howtogeek.com/428
337/not-all-5g-is-equal-
millimeter-wave-low-band-and-
mid-band-explained/

Johnson, J. (2018, October 23).
    *Countless Studies Show 5G
    Frequencies Cause Illness.*
    Retrieved from EMF TESTS:
    http://emftests.com/countless-
    studies-show-5g-frequencies-
    cause-illness/
Lung Institute. (2016, January 29). *5
    Tips to Increase your Blood
    Oxygen Naturally.* Retrieved
    from Lung Institue Breath Easier:
    https://lunginstitute.com/blog/5-
    tips-to-increase-your-blood-
    oxygen-naturally-2/
McPhilips, E. (2015, June 24). *Hearing
    Loss and Infrasound, Can You
    Hear It?* Retrieved from
    Audicus:
    https://www.audicus.com/hearing
    -loss-and-infrasound/
Miller, R. (2003, March 3). *SYNTHETIC
    TELEPATHY AND THE EARLY
    MIND WARS* .
Moskowitz, J. (2019, October 17). *We
    Have No Reason to Believe 5G Is
    Safe.* Retrieved from Scientific
    American:
    https://blogs.scientificamerican.c
    om/observations/we-have-no-
    reason-to-believe-5g-is-safe/

Nandan, R. &. (2014). ANALYSIS OF MOBILE PHONE RADIATIONS. *International Journal of Advanced Research in Electronics and Communication Engineering.*

National Research Nuclear University. (2016, October 12). *Scientists research effects of infrasonic vibrations in humans.* Retrieved from National Research Nuclear University: https://m.phys.org/news/2016-10-scientists-effects-infrasonic-vibrations-humans.html

Neurohealth. (2020). *The Science of Brainwaves.* Retrieved from Neurohealth: https://nhahealth.com/brainwaves-the-language/

NTD. (2019, June 4). *NTD News.* Retrieved from Doctors call for delaying deployment of 5G Due to Health Risks: https://www.youtube.com/watch?v=-T2R2htAaqg&feature=youtu.be&fbclid=IwAR2j8w0WInfl9ZQdyIZC7XVl_urCSpMeqLSzN9f0VoguUBnuxbSV4JE1ilw

Pretz, K. (2019, November 12). *Will 5G Be Bad for Our Health?* Retrieved from I EEE SPECTRUM: https://spectrum.ieee.org/news-from-around-ieee/the-institute/ieee-member-news/will-5g-be-bad-for-our-health

Rejuvinea Health. (2014). *How to Oxygenate Your Body.* Retrieved from Rejuvinea Health: http://werejuvenate.com/how-to-oxygenate-your-body/

Schomburg, T. (2014, October 23). *How to Heal Your Body by Using the Frequency of Life.* Retrieved from Meducated Org : https://medium.com/meducated-org/how-to-heal-your-body-by-using-the-frequency-of-life-9307af550fbb

Segan, S. (2020, January 2). *What Is 5G?* Retrieved from PC Magazine: https://www.pcmag.com/news/what-is-5g

Shinde, A. (2020). *3 Breathing Exercises to Fight Stress and Raise Oxygen Levels.* Retrieved from Aging Care: https://www.agingcare.com/articl

es/breathing-exercises-decrease-stress-and-raise-oxygen-levels-189489.htm

Silva, J. (2020). *Low and normal blood oxygen levels: What to know.* Retrieved from Medical News Today: https://www.medicalnewstoday.com/articles/321044#measuring-blood-oxygen-levels

Tandy, V. (1998). The Ghost in the Machine. *Published in the Journal of the Society for Psychical Research.*

Vaidyanatha, V. (2018). *What Are Microwave Weapons? US Diplomats In China, Cuba Likely Victims.* Retrieved from International Business Times.

Vincent, B. (2020, March 25). *White House Releases National Strategy for 5G Security.* Retrieved from Nextgov: https://www.nextgov.com/emerging-tech/2020/03/white-house-releases-national-strategy-5g-security/164109/

Wagner, P. (2020, January 9). *How to Protect Yourself from 5G and EMF Radiation.* Retrieved from GAIA:

https://www.gaia.com/article/how-to-protect-yourself-from-5g-and-emf-radiation

Westall, S. (2020, February). *Court Rules: 5G Danger is Not a Conspiracy w/ Mark Steele.* Retrieved from Business Game Changers with Sarah Westall.

Whitehawk, L. (2018). *HUSO.* Retrieved from How Does Sound Frequency Heal Us?

World Health Organization. (2019, November 7). *Electromagnetic fields (EMF).* Retrieved from World Health Organization: https://www.who.int/peh-emf/about/WhatisEMF/en/index1.html

Yoder, P. L. (2017). Totally Booked Practice. In P. Yoder, *Totally Booked Practice.*

Made in USA - Kendallville, IN
1086683_9798636982647